Have
Confidence

Alankrita

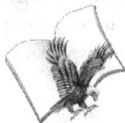

V&S PUBLISHERS

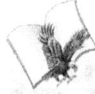

Published by:

V&S PUBLISHERS

F-2/16, Ansari Road, Daryaganj, New Delhi-110002
☎ 011-23240026, 011-23240027 • *Fax:* 011-23240028
Email: info@vspublishers.com • *Website:* www.vspublishers.com

Branch : Hyderabad
5-1-707/1, Brij Bhawan (Beside Central Bank of India Lane)
Bank Street, Koti, Hyderabad - 500 095
☎ 040-24737290
E-mail: vspublishershyd@gmail.com

Branch Office : Mumbai
Jaywant Industrial Estate, 2nd Floor–222, Tardeo Road
Opposite Sobo Central Mall, Mumbai – 400 034
☎ 022-23510736
E-mail: vspublishersmum@gmail.com

Follow us on: **t** **f** **in**

All books available at **www.vspublishers.com**

Preface

Amidst 6 billion people in the world there are only a handful of men and women who are able to achieve greatness. They create epochs, author the annals of history, discover new worlds and pioneer novel concepts. These men and women come to control the destinies of millions and give new dimensions to human existence. They carry attributes that are responsible for making life great. These may be either mental qualities or the qualities of heart, body or soul. This book is a humble attempt to identify the persons who possessed some of such qualities. If one reads it, it is certain that he/she will gather the self-confidence which is absolutely required to lead a good life.

Whatever may be our endowments, background, situation or time, we must try our level best to comprehend and nurture our true potential. Why not explore it?

Here we commence a breathtaking journey towards building a world of HAVE CONFIDENCE.

☐☐

Contents

Preface   *3*

Chapter One

JOURNEY TOWARDS SELF-CONFIDENCE

• The Benchmark of Greatness   7
• Breaking the Inertia   15
• Forming a Mini-Universe Within   18
• Inspirations   21
• Translating Ideas into Life   23

Chapter Two

CULTIVATING SELF-CONFIDENCE

• The Psychic Influence at Birth   26
• The Years of Adolescence   28
• Always a Winner!   34

Chapter Three

STRATEGY FOR BUILDING CONFIDENCE

• Prioritizing   37
• Planning   40
• Time Scheduling   41
• The Significance of Motivation   42

Chapter One

Journey Towards Self-confidence

The Benchmark of Greatness

If a man hasn't discovered something
that he will die for, he isn't fit to live.
— Martin Luther-I

These words are as stirring and true as the life of its believer. In a few words, the very meaning of human existence has been summed up. Life is nothing more than a search - a continuous search for a cause to live and die to be governed by the thoughts and dreams and propelled by a concealed urge to achieve Greatness. In this vast sea of humanity, let us take a solemn pledge - a pledge to accomplish that for which we are born, to conquer our follies and failings and stand apart from the teeming millions, as the one who leaves his footprints for others to walk upon. But before we commence our journey towards greatness, we must contemplate upon its nature and try to find a coherence with it in our own short life.

Defining Greatness

Greatness can be termed as the measurement of the 'intrinsic value' of a person or his deeds. Greatness is never tainted with selfish motives. Rather, it is guided by a strong motive which is the 'welfare' of mankind. A man can earn lots of money, build palaces, provide the best to his family and wallow in the swamp of glory, but can't reach greatness if his efforts are guided only towards self elevation. On the other hand, a soldier fighting for his country after putting everything at stake or a modest social worker dedicating his life for social upliftment without caring for his personal well-being, can definitely be termed as Great. Greatness has within its bosom, the central theme of "Giving" - giving knowledge, cultivating faith, giving solace, giving peace and above all giving up yourself for the good of others.

It has been truly said by Khalel Gibran -

You give but little when you give of your possessions. It is when you give of yourself that you truly give.

The benchmark of GREATNESS comprises the following virtues:

• *Possessing a worthwhile cause*

In the words of Swami Vivekananda **"Life is short, Give up to a great cause."** It is only when a person rises above his own petty self and dedicates himself to a cause, that he sows the seeds of an enlightened life. He becomes an embodiment of an ideology and gradually loses his own tiny existence. This is the first benchmark towards greatness. He and his cause become one. The cause can be social, moral or patriotic.

One such man was Martin Luther. On October 31, 1517, when Martin Luther was nailing his thesis upon the door of the church at Wittenburg, criticizing the sale of indulgences, never did he realize that he was going to give birth to a new religious sect called the **Protestants.** Amidst turbulent opposition from the greatest powers in Europe, he kept his cause glowing like a radiant sun. What kept him moving was his unflinching faith in his cause which he believed was the voice of his conscience.

I can and will retract nothing, as it is dangerous to act against one's conscience was his confident proclamation. Martin Luther was quick to recognize the spiritual fervour within him. He was grossly unsatisfied with religious abuses doled out by the priests. His strong religious convictions grew into a rage and he threw his entire life to the Reformation of Christianity. His contributions to religion helped to transform the medieval world into the modern.

- *Driven by a single obsession*

    Great men and women always live with "one mission". Their minds are filled by an obsession to accomplish their mission. They are never daunted by circumstances or conditions, rather their eyes are fixed upon what they desire to achieve. Day and night, their thoughts revolve around their mission.

    In ancient India, a little before the battle **Mahabharata** was fought, sage *Dronacharya* was assigned the task of teaching archery to his disciples–young princes of *Hastinapur* among whom the name of *Arjuna* stands apart. As a young boy, he had only one obsession - to be the world's greatest archer. One fine afternoon, all the princes were asked to aim at the eye of a clay bird. To test their concentration, Dronacharya enquired all the princes "What do you all see?" Some princes pointed towards the trees, the surroundings, some towards the well and the river. It was only Arjun who said "I only see the bird's eye." The surroundings made no effect on him, for he had just one thing in his mind - his goal of becoming the greatest archer of the world.

    Our Ancient history stands as a testimony to the fact that our country has produced so many great archers but none can match the stature of Arjun.

- *Unchanging conviction*

    Swami Vivekananda puts it very aptly "**I will drink the ocean, to preserve soul. Mountains will crumble into dust at my feet**". Such men of great mettle erect a fortress of strong and unmoving conviction around themselves which none can pierce. They always live with the feeling that they are born to accomplish some great task. For them, it is the cause that matters and not the condition.

One such hero was David Livingstone - the man who accorded respect and knowledge to the Dark Continent of Africa. Amidst the negative pursuits of his father, the dangerous journeys across Africa, the physical dual with a lion in which he almost lost his left arm and the ailing health of his children, he crossed the insurmountable Kalahari Desert and discovered numerous unknown rivers like the Zouga, Zambezi, and lands like Landa in Central Africa. He was nearly crippled with fever, ill-health, lack of food and equipment but he continued his adventures until he became a hero. Eventually he died in the lap of the mysterious continent of Africa.

Nothing could daunt him.... not even death for he continued to live in the hearts of millions of adventure lovers around the world. Africa definitely owes a never-ending debt to him.

- ### Consistent labour

And thou wilt give thyself relief, if thou doest every act of thy life, as if it were the last

–Marcus Aurelius

We must work in such a way towards our mission as if every moment is the last moment of our life. Great people reap the fruits of their incessant labour. Their only concern is towards the work which they undertake without thinking of its results. They are always guided by the 'spirit of action' and not by the jugglery of words. Hence the most appropriate way to achieve greatness is to "burn the midnight lamp" both literally as well as figuratively and continue working towards the attainment of the cause.

Therefore one of the **Upanishads,** the sacred Hindu

texts, echoes with these powerful words:

Arise, Awake and stop not till the goal is reached.

When passivity takes to labour - actions take place. Peter the Great of Russia was a raw and uncivilized ruler of a mighty empire. He set out to study, acquire knowledge and make himself appropriate for his empire. "Myself a pupil, I seek teachers", was a seal that he carried with himself.

He acquired immense knowledge and returned to his native place Russia for initiating the process of westernization and reforms. Russia at that time had no navy and seaports. Peter was determined to establish both.

In 1695, Peter made his first attack upon Azov but was utterly defeated. But he was committed to his plans. He made another attempt. This time he met with convincing success. With this success, he poured in large sums of money to maintain a fleet of ships in the waters that he had conquered.

Two years later, he sent a large number of Russians to Holland, England, Italy and Germany to acquire knowledge about civilizations. He himself studied Architecture, Mechanics, Fortification, Printing, Anatomy and Astronomy in Holland. His labour continued.

From Holland, he went to England where he learnt the theory and practice of ship-building. Apart from this, he gave his mind to many new things such as setting up universities, hospitals, Royal societies, cathedrals and churches in his country for which he visited all these in England.

Not only this, Peter also toiled in shipyards as an apprentice to learn about naval establishments and dockyards.

Although Peter had many vices, his energy was boundless. He undertook the biggest and the smallest tasks with the equal amount of ease. All his drawbacks could somehow be compensated with his extreme hard-work.

He exhausted himself in the endeavour to build up his country. He took up the responsibility of transforming a semi-Asiatic state into one of the most developed regions of Europe. His efforts bore fruit because of his consistent labour.

- ### *Devoid of evil inclines*

All great men have one thing in common - their love for humanity and their hatred for evil. Before venturing out for a mission "clean up your soul" and submit yourself to a life of goodness. If you fail to conquer evil, you will certainly fail to enter the kingdom of the great. Every great movement which has flourished on the earth, has been triggered off by the "essence of nobility". The re-nowned dictum "From log cabin to Whitehouse" sums up the entire life of Abraham Lincoln. A poor nomad born in a log cabin, lost his mother at an early age, hit hard by the humiliations of slavery and facing tough attacks from the US press, Abraham Lincoln went on to become one of the greatest men, US has ever produced - conquering the hearts of millions of people with his sense of justice and sincerity. His ascent to the post of the President of USA was not of as much significance as his notable contributions in the field of social justice and the abolition of slavery and amendment of the Constitution of America. His life echoed with one principle - the benefit of mankind.

"I have done nothing to make any Human being remember that I have lived. Yet what I wish to live for is to connect my name with the events of my day and generation, to link my name with some-

thing which will be of interest to my fellow-men," said Abraham Lincoln

This was written when he was a young man of thirty-two. He had more misery in life than happiness. Once while he was trying to come out of a fit of depression, he strongly felt like committing suicide. This man could not have asked for more as from a poor man, born in a log cabin, he rose to become the President of the United States of America. His life is almost an epic of U.S.A which almost owes him today, its existence as a Nation.

Born on 12th February, 1809 in Kentucky, Abraham was the son of a wandering carpenter. He was fascinated by the greenery and far away lands. At the age of four, Abraham began his wanderings along with his family. His father, being extremely restless moved to Indiana. For one year, the family had to live in floorless, half-built camp made up of uncut logs. Life was extremely difficult as the region was swampy. Animals did not thrive and human beings began falling victims to Malaria. While facing hardships, Abraham lost his mother on account of a fatal disease. After the death of his mother, family began to wander to distant lands. It was then that Abraham, for the first time saw his step mother. A new life began for Abraham. His new mother insisted that he should go to school. Abraham, known as Abe, began his educational career in fits and starts. He learnt some reading and writing. But from that day onwards he began to read everything that came on his way. He grew up into a strong man but was known for his eccentricity for he talked on various topics and tried to imitate preachers and orators.

The turning point in his life came in 1828 when for the first time he was exposed to the outside world infested with slavery. He began his career by carrying agricultural produce to New Orleans by boat. It gave him the opportunity to study the condition of Negro slaves. He was moved to see their appalling condition.

Abraham Lincoln found the mission of his life. He decided to abolish slavery from America. His journey towards Greatness commenced when he chose a mission that would alleviate the condition of the Blacks.

Later on, Abraham Lincoln became the manager of the store where he used to sell his agricultural products. There he engaged himself in extensive reading as well as in local politics by acting as a clerk of the local polls.

Being the scholar of the district, he became a participator in local political debates and was drawn in towards politics. But due to his interest in politics, he almost became insolvent in his store business. But he continued his involvement with politics.

Abraham Lincoln became the candidate for the Legislature in the year 1834. But another pursuit caught his interest during those days. It was law. Abraham formed a law partnership firm with William H. Herndon who later became his biographer.

An address that he gave in New York gave him a nation-wide reputation. People were surprised to see that an uncouth, ill-clad, lanky lawyer had the power to sway the masses. The press began to attack him severely. He was termed as a "third-rate country lawyer, with poor grammar, clumsy jokes, gorilla like looks and a shabby dressing sense". The slave owning aristocrats despised him. But he became popular among the masses for whom he was fighting.

Abraham Lincoln met with one misfortune after another. One of the gravest among them was the bad relations with his wife and the illness of both his sons. But amidst all these problems, Abraham Lincoln never hesitated from signing a proclamation for the complete emancipation of the slaves.

Finally after umpteen trials and tribulations, Abraham Lincoln succeeded in accomplishing the mission of his life - the thirteenth amendment bill was passed and the Constitution of the United States of America was amended. Slavery was abolished from USA.

Finally, on April 14, 1865, Abraham Lincoln assumed the highest post in the land. He was elected as the President of the country.

His sense of Equality, deep-rooted benevolence, forgiveness and faith in Justice ensured his sublime greatness.

He possessed a great sagacity to guiding people through the tumults of mighty revolutions with the help of deep religiosity, an admirable singleness of purpose, a flaming passion to free his country from the bonds of slavery. It was a luminous example of utmost honesty and purity, the possession of keen and inexplicable magnetism and the moderation in temperament that made him soothing to his subordinates.

Abraham Lincoln was the architect of his own destiny. He rose with every opportunity, conquered every crisis, performed every duty. Civilization will hold his name in eternal renown as a patriot, leader and liberator. He truly possessed Supreme confidence which provided him best opportunities in life.

Breaking the Inertia

Building "Self-confidence" is not a day's work. It needs years and years of dedication, perseverance and patience. But good work can only be done if the thoughts are moulded accordingly. To mould our thoughts into a perfect cast, it is necessary for us to let loose our imagination till they crystallize into a specific pattern.

Now, what is inertia and how can we break it?

Inertia, in this context, is nothing but the inability to break loose.

Since our very childhood, *we are afraid to dream, to imagine and to allow our thoughts to break free*. The reasons for this can be many. Let us discuss some of them:

The first and foremost cause of inertia is *Insecurity*.

Insecurity

Every person possesses an insecurity regarding his sustenance. How will I maintain my livelihood? How will I meet my family's expenses? are the common concerns of one and all although these concerns are quite genuine. A person must learn the art of making his survival interests, a part of his mission and not vice-versa. Try to take out a middle path between your family responsibilities and your mission.

Trample Upon Insecurity

All great people have had difficulties in fulfilling their family needs, but they never undermined their zeal. Karl Marx (whom we shall discuss later) was confronted by extreme penury. He found it difficult to meet his both ends. His family reeled under poverty. But he gave to the world one of the greatest movements for the betterment of the poor and downtrodden.

Sacrifice yourself for the family, the family for the neighbourhood, the neighbourhood for the city, the city for the state, the state for the country and the country for Humanity. For there is no duty on this earth which comes above Humanity.

- *Family pressure*

  The second major cause of our mental inertia is family pressure. It might be possible that one wants to become a great musician but his parents want him to become a doctor. In this case, what will he like to do?

- *Never succumb to pressure*

    If one strongly believes that he possesses the aptitude of becoming a great musician, then he must not succumb to pressure. One should stick to one's aim and be truthful to it. One must have faith in one's convictions and then proceed. On the other hand, if he succumbs to pressure against his own will, he will neither be able to do justice to his profession nor to his parents. He will remain half-hearted towards his profession and unhappy with his parents. One must be confident about what he desires to achieve in life.

Lack of Confidence

Lack of confidence is also a significant reason for allowing our thinking to break loose. If one feels that he is having the potential of becoming a TV Artist and wants to render information, knowledge and entertainment to people across the country, the only thing which would impede him would be lack of confidence.

- *Nurture the confidence*

    Confidence is like a plant - it needs to be manured, watered and exposed before sunlight. It needs the manure of a mission, the water of continuous self-persuasion and exposed to the sunlight of skills and hardwork.

    We have to work hard with our thoughts as well as our confidence and at no moment in our life, allow it to perish. The quality of the plant depends upon the quality of the soil, similarly the quality of our work will directly depend upon the quality of our thoughts. So fill your mind with the greatest thoughts and out of that will emerge great work.

    Once you overcome the impediments that come in way of our thoughts, you must unleash the forces of your mind. Release your creative imagination and aim for the highest. The amount of efforts that are needed for survival are no less than the amount of endeavours required to become great. Then why settle for something less. Greatness is just a matter of attitude, perceptions and implementation. Give vent to your thoughts–aim for the highest.

Napoleon once said, "Forty centuries are looking down upon you. So March on! It is the spirit which works and not the hands. Break yourself free from the crippling influence of "inertia".

It is never a sin to dream.

Never hesitate to dream. Always keep them sublime and keep in mind that you have to follow your dreams till their fulfilment. Let not your thoughts become a victim of inertia.

Going Against Usual Norms

No great work has ever been accomplished without opposition. If going against systems is a sin then every great social and spiritual leader is a sinner. If you have to break certain norms for the betterment of mankind and for the fulfilment of your noble mission, go ahead–the Divine grace will bestow His choicest blessings upon you.

If you are still contemplating, your doubts will be certainly put to rest, once you fortify your thoughts - let's see how.

Forming a Mini-Universe Within

Once you have broken your "inertia" and "dared to dream" about your mission, you have already commenced your journey towards greatness. Now the next thing which you are required to do is to "fortify" your thoughts. To make sure that whatever dream you are nurturing within remains with you till its final accomplishment. How can you do that?

Our mind is divided into three portions - the conscious, the sub-conscious and the super-conscious. The last i.e. super-conscious is only active in men who attain divinity. So, we are only concerned with the first two. Fill your conscious mind with thoughts about your mission by perpetual contemplation. What is perpetual contemplation? It involves:

Self Persuasion

Persuade yourself constantly by reading motivational literature, gaining knowledge about the ways and means of achieving your mission and also by nurturing your thoughts in the same direction.

- *Fixing your ideal*

  You should begin with fixing up such a person as your ideal who has already reached the zenith of the field you intend to pursue. Try to study his life in detail. Search for the qualities he or she possessed. Try to learn from the mistakes which he committed. It will help you frame-up your own future image and enhance your confidence level.

- *Perpetual contemplation on your aim*

  After waking up in the morning, repeat your aim several times. Abstain from loose thinking that can distract you from your path.

- *Let each day be another step*

  Our entire life is a ladder and each day is a step towards the top of the ladder. Hence do not waste a single moment. At the end of each day, you should feel that you have taken another step towards your mission.

  You can try out a game. Keep 365 coins with you in reserve. Let each coin represent a day. If you feel that you haven't fully utilized the day, take one coin out from the reserve fund and put it away. In case you feel that you have outdone your day's target- add 25 cents to the fund. At the end of every week, month and year, calculate your reserves. You will be able to measure the worth of time in tangible terms.

Try to form a Universe within you, which remains fortified. In order to create this Mini Universe as well as to fortify it, you need a very strong defence mechanism. Defend the boundaries of your Universe with a strong General - your "conscience". Your conscience must keep a check on every outside element (thought) that enters your Universe as well as departs from it. The only thing that should be borne in mind is never to disturb the harmonious balance that pertains in your mini-universe.

If this mini-universe is your mind, then there are surely distractors or impediments, who are waiting to destroy your equilibrium. Let us see which are those distractors that can harm your Universe.

Conditions

Conditions in life will keep varying from time to time. Try to remain balanced under every condition. For that, you must have strong faith in your mission. Secondly, you must pray regularly because prayer helps you to develop faith and enhance your internal strength. Prayer will help you to protect your mini-universe from all vagaries of the external world.

- *Discouragement*

   If you get daunted because of discouragement, it proves that somehow or the other you are still lacking faith in your own mission. The person who believes in himself, nothing can affect him adversely.

- *Depression*

    Another problem which you may face very often is that of depression. While pursuing the aims, one may be confronted with innumerable problems. The problems can be multifarious - of health, of money, of social acceptance or of family uncertainties. These difficulties are a part of any great mission. It is like a plant of rose whose beauty gets accentuated by the presence of thorns. No great work has ever been achieved without hurdles. Hence, whatever problems come your way they must be dealt sportingly without letting the devil of depression win. Depression not only reduces the level of motivation, it also saps out vital energy from your mind and body. Let us consider now how to tackle the problem of depression.

- *Tackle the problem of depression*

    - Always try to strike the problem at the root.
    - Try to take your mind away from the depressing factor and focus it on different activities.
    - Take some time off from ponderous work schedules and relax.
    - Practise some mild breathing exercises, like slow inhalation and exhalation.
    - Repeat regularly to yourself, "Nobody can shatter my confidence."

    Always protect your mini-universe against all odds, because within that tiny world rests your entire future....... Let us consider now the value of inspiration in building Self-confidence.

Inspirations

The dream that man weaves is always woven with the help of inspirations. These inspirations can either be derived from great events or great experiences, but these dreams certainly become the yardstick of a man's character. We all possess an uncanny knack of learning from inspiring factors and events. But we must not overlook small incidents or even insignificant beings who are inspiring us every moment.

Let us begin with the 5 elements of Nature that have been the continuous source of inspiration for mankind since eternity. We are all made up of these five elements and we are ultimately going to blend into all of them. So why not derive certain inspirations from them!

Air

Air is the source of survival of every living animal on the earth. It keeps an equal eye upon the rich and the poor, the famous and the notorious or the high class and the low class. Its message for humanity is that of "Equanimity".

Fire

Fire can give life as well as take life. It depends upon how we use it. It is neither a friend nor a foe. Rather it is a thing to be used prudently. If utilized properly, it can give us food and energy and if handled carelessly, it can cause us injury and devastation.

Water

Water possesses the unique attribute of perpetuity. Whatever the conditions might be, water can never remain still. It keeps moving from one place to another. Its velocity depends upon various factors but its movement is never affected. It can never be broken, cut or destroyed. Its flexibility makes it ever existent.

Earth

Since millions of years, man has trampled upon earth yet she has been silently bearing every deed of man. She possesses the extremes of endurance and patience for the fulfilment of her mission - helping mankind to survive.

People who are desirous of achieving their mission in life must imbibe endurance and patience like mother earth. In that case, she is the greatest source of man's inspiration.

Sky (Ether)

Why is the sky so significant? It is important because it gives mankind the idea of vastness. It is the crown of the Lord which never comes to an end.

Another synonym of life is 'expansion'. In the words of Swami Vivekananda, **"Expansion is life, contraction is death"**. Never restrict your thinking, let it grow till it encompasses the entire humanity. "Keep growing till you are able to provide shelter to all those who are beneath you." This is one of the keys for unlocking the treasure of 'greatness' and self-confidence.

Translating Ideas into Life

It is true that if a new idea clicks, it can turn an ordinary man into a genius. The man who discovered the idea of gravity was none other than the great Newton who churned out a brilliant idea from a small incidence like the falling of an apple. His main achievement was to discover the concept of 'gravity', which we made it known to the entire humankind. This simple thought which struck his mind required years of tenacious research. When it got converted into life, it made an ordinary farm boy, one of the greatest scientists the world has ever produced. If he did not possess the capability of converting dreams into ideas, he would have remained anonymous and insignificant throughout his life like millions of other farmers of his age and time.

Ideas lose their significance till they are translated into life. Every single idea needs to be planted, first in the mind and then on the ground.

Now the question arises - how to translate ideas into life?

Let us take it step by step.

Step One

Prepare a Plan

Before you begin to translate ideas into life, you must possess a clear conception of what you actually desire to do. For that, you must have a clear-cut plan before yourself. The plan must be tangible, quantified and scheduled. Without a proper plan your journey towards greatness will become as aimless as a rudderless ship which is oblivious of its destination.

Step Two

Make a Schedule

Once the plan is ready, you should then discreetly divide it into 3 phases. The present, the immediate future and the future.

Whatever is mentioned in the immediate future, it must be taken up in the right earnest. It must be implemented in your day to day life.

Just one thing must be clearly underlined in your mind. Never take up any profession, just for the sake of maintaining your livelihood - if it is not in concomitance to your ultimate mission. It will not only sap out your precious time and energy, but will also lead to your deviation from the final goal.

Step Three

Revise your Plan

For the success in any task, it is necessary to revise the plan on time. So at the end of every week, try to analyze your progress towards your ultimate mission. See if you have moved even an inch towards your destination. You may also review your strategies from a time to time basis. However, every task should be time-bound so that you are compelled to fulfil your targets. The fulfilment of small commitments will give you the taste of success. This itself will be a major motivator for you in your journey towards success.

Step Four

Association with like minded people

In our journey towards greatness, we must be very careful regarding the kind of people we meet. You should avoid the company of those who are not supportive to your mission. You should also avoid friction with others because that spoils your mental peace and eventually leads to failure.

Besides following the above steps, a few other things are also necessary to follow. Among them are: Independence of thought and action. Human beings as well as animals cherish independence. Persons who are dependant on others for success may face 'dejection' - if that person does not accomplish the task given to him, 'dissatisfaction'- if he falls short of expectations and 'deceit' - if he is betrayed by the other on account of greed, jealousy or vindication. Hence independence of thought and action is necessary in order to insure man from all the three D's.

After winning over the three D's, you are ready to march towards greatness. But before marching forward, it is absolutely necessary to take a quick dip into the past. To know about the cherished deeds of great men and women, to analyze the mistakes that man had committed and also to choose the precious gems of wisdom from the greatest events in human history.

❑❑

Chapter Three

Cultivating Self-confidence

*"I think somehow we learn who we really are
and then live with that decision."*

F.D. Roosevelt

The Psychic Influence at Birth

It is very true that whatever we achieve in life is directly based upon what we think since our very inception. This process of grasping facts from the external environment, analyzing those facts and eventually assimilating them within us begins even before our birth. Science reveals that the child begins to form attributes even when he is in the womb of his mother. That is why pregnant women are advised not to see violence, vulgarity or anything which is immoral. Rather they should engage themselves in reading good books and scriptures, and in prayer and devotion and with the activities that are moral and warranted. We are bound to reap what we sow.

Can we expect to get mangoes by sowing the seeds of grapes? It is never possible. Therefore, the parents have to be extremely careful with the upbringing of their children especially during the first 5 years of the child's life. If the foundation becomes strong, the future may be ensured.

The attributes of fear, insecurity, lust and anger begin to sprout up right from the first couple of years.

At the time of birth, the child is tied up with the umbilical cord of the mother. While actually coming into this world, the child is separated from the mother simply by cutting this cord. This is for the first time that the child undergoes the act of pain. if the doctor is not careful and the pain is little sharp, the child is bound to develop traces of fear. Such children are more insecure as compared to the others.

The second factor, which proves to be instrumental in moulding the psyche of children, is his upbringing in the first three years. It has been seen that children who are breastfed are more secure and healthy as compared to children who are not. Hence, it is natural for the child to experience the closeness of his mother before opening his eyes. It is also quite true that children till the age of 3 are most receptive to new things. They tend to grasp almost everything, which they see or feel. During this phase, the children must be exposed to colours, natural beauty and acts of kindness such as feeding and patting animals, caressing younger brothers and sisters, sharing toys etc. People who are destined to achieve greatness exhibit a keen sense of enquiry and sensitivity at this age. These are the formative and educative years for a child, which most elders tend to overlook. Children who are overtly protected grow up to be timid. On the other hand children who are not given ample care become harsh and sometimes insensitive to others.

Children till the age of 5 have a highly emotive nature. They are very much aware of their surroundings. The relationship between parents proves to be a vital factor in the mental and emotional make-up of a child. Parents who are always quarrelling bitterly in front of their child are directly responsible for spoiling the child's future. Therefore, it is absolutely necessary for a child to get a cordial ambience where he can bloom.

Children are extremely sensitive to sounds and pictures. Blaring noise and loud sounds can adversely affect the mind of the child. He can become mentally weak, irritable and sometimes even violent. Viewing vulgar movies and pictures can also have a detrimental effect on the mind of a child. Mothers who expose themselves to the electronic media during pregnancy may ruin the general health and mental make-up of the child.

From birth to adolescence, the best school is the mother's lap. The child should not be sent to school till the age of 5, instead he should be encouraged to be with nature and discover the world with his own eyes. This concept of *discovering by one's self*, needs encouragement and due implementation. As we have discussed before, nature is indeed the best teacher. If we want to learn about the birds and the bees, what better place can we find other than the lap of nature?

Hence, during and after the birth of a child, he must be kept away from the following:

- *Noise*
- *Pollution*
- *Violence*
- *Media and*
- *Computers*

The child should be exposed more and more to the following:

- *Colours*
- *Plants & Trees*
- *Birds & Animals*
- *Devotional songs*
- *Fresh Air*

If infancy is well managed, the child is almost ready to welcome adolescence.

The Years of Adolescence

The years between 10 and 17 are the most significant years of a person's life. The period of adolescence as it is called, is the formative period, when man can either make his life or break his life. During these years, a youngster is full of zest and energy. If this energy is not given the right direction, it tends to lose its way. The energy needs an outlet - either by way of physical activities or by way of mental activities. When the students start complaining of pressure and work-load, their problem needs to be eased out with the help of sports, various types of performing arts, mass communication and social activities. It is indeed very difficult for individuals to change the education system or even avoid it, but it is always possible to carve out a parallel stream of education for the healthy development of the child.

This brings us to the question - *What kind of education is required for imbibing the virtues of greatness?*

The Ideal Education

In the words of Swami Vivekananda **Education is not the amount of information that is stuffed into your brains and runs riot there all through your life. Education must be man making and character building.**

Education is quite distinct from literacy. Merely by cramming up facts and figures, a man cannot call himself educated. It is better to instil five virtues and to live upon them with heart and soul than to learn by heart almost a whole library. If we look into the lives of great men and women, we will find that it is not bookish knowledge that has made them great. Rather it is their experience and understanding of truth that has made them great. There have been innumerable people who did not get the opportunity to get higher education, but their whole life was rich and colourful because of their rich experience and other qualities. One such person was James Watt.

James Watt

The harnessing of the steam power has been one of the

greatest inventions in the field of science and the man who brought about this great invention is none other than James Watt.

As a child he showed no potential and his indolence annoyed his parents. At the tea table his aunt used to chide saying, "James, I never saw such an idle boy as you are; take a book or employ yourself usefully; for the last hour you have not spoken one word, but taken off the lid of the kettle and put it on again, holding now a cup and now a silver spoon over the steam, watching how it rises from the sprout, catching and counting the drops it falls into." Later it was proved by the scientists that as he intently poured his thoughts on the boiling kettle and the steam, he was actually working on the theory of *Thermodynamics.*

Watt kept on observing, discussing and contemplating on facts. One Sunday morning, while he was taking his constitutional after church, he hit upon a great idea which made him the father of the Industrial Revolution. The boiler was too small to operate an engine; therefore the engine was wasteful in the consumption of steam. The solution was to produce an engine consuming less steam.

James Watt was known for his unfailing concentration. He knew how to stick to a particular task over an extended period of time till he got the results. Not only this, he was also inclined towards humanitarian considerations. James Watt refused to develop his engine by the use of high-pressure steam. He thought that it would endanger public life by causing explosions.

Till the end of his life, he continued his obsession for inventions. He stuck to whatever he thought. And that became the reason for his success.

Rabindra Nath Tagore:
The Epitome of Education

The Wakeful ageless God Calls today on our soul- the

soul that is measureless, the soul that is undefeated, the soul that is destined to immortality and yet today the soul that lies in the dust.

These few lines written by Tagore show the exaltation of his thoughts, the essence of his spirit and the truth of present conditions. In these lines, he has in fact given the wisdom of the entire world.

Rabindra Nath Tagore was born on May 6, 1861 in Bengal in an elite Hindu Family. He was the youngest son in his family. During his childhood, he was brought up with discipline. But all attempts to send him to school failed. Rabindra Nath felt choked in the confines of school. He felt that it cramped his spirit of independence, his creativity and imagination. He enjoyed studying in the natural beauty of his garden, which infused a sense of serenity and harmony. Private lessons were imparted to him at home. He came in contact with cultured, thoughtful and educated people who were close family acquaintances.

Once as a small boy, he went to the Himalayas along with his father. The soothing atmosphere and the close company of his learned father intensified his sympathetic and mystical temperament. The early knowledge of the **Upanishads** that he received from his father made him develop a spirit of Universal love and brotherhood. His elder brothers and women in the family gave him ample encouragement in developing Self-confidence.

On September 20, 1877, he went to England for the first time with the purpose of studying Law. He returned to Bengal with novel ideas in religion, literature and politics. Rabindra Nath's strong upbringing made him evolve a highly imaginative, sublime and thoughtful mind. He composed some of the best poetry of all times.

The year 1901 was the milestone in his life. It saw the foundation of Shantiniketan, an International University on the lines of forest schools or **Gurukuls** of Ancient India. The idea was to expose the students to natural surroundings instead of closed confinements and to enable them to develop a free and universal spirit. He strongly believed in the inculcation of creativity and mysticism instead of a cold and calculative mind. Here in his school he wanted to develop perfect world citizens.

In 1903, Rabindra Nath was awarded the Nobel Prize for **Gitanjali**. Later on, it was followed by his knighthood. But due to the Jallianwala Bagh massacre in 1919, Rabindra Nath Tagore, exhibiting sublime love for his country, relinquished his knighthood.

Rabindra Nath Tagore gave the message of extreme compassion, tolerance, universality and patriotism to the world. His greatness lies in the fact that his childhood and adolescence were utilized in gaining true knowledge alloyed with the gems of supreme spirituality and openness.

The years between eleven to seventeen are extremely important for every individual. This is the period when a person undergoes many physical, mental and emotional changes. An adolescent must be dealt with extreme care for from this stage onwards, he can either go towards the heights of success and glory or fall into the abyss of ruin and destruction. Therefore, it is necessary to know about the problems during adolescence.

Problems During Adolescence

During adolescence a child can face various problems. This is the period when a boy or a girl steps into the threshold of adulthood. The child undergoes immense emotional turbulence. It is during this period that the raw energies must be converted into creative activities. The emphasis should be on the holistic development of the child rather than on academic development only.

The problems generally faced are complexities, evil company, feeling of inferiority or lack of confidence and sometimes superiority complex.

Complexities

Complexities arise when a person becomes conscious of what others think or feel about him. Instead of concentrating on his work, he begins to concentrate on others. Children who lack a proper family, sound guidance and care, develop certain negative complexities whereas children who are too much pampered, develop a positive complex. Both types of complexities can undermine the progress of an individual.

This can be elaborated further. Complexities are of two kinds:

Inferiority & Lack of Confidence

Inferiority complex can be dangerous for a growing individual. Such a person can never work towards greatness. He often commits mistakes in order to hide his own weaknesses.

Superiority Complex

Superiority complex is basically an over-estimation of the self. It can arise because of good looks, earnings, learning or family. A person suffering from superiority complex actually restricts his scope to grow. He begins to feel that he has something more than others. Such people become unpopular among friends and relatives. Although they can feel happy at times, it can never give everlasting joy. Such a complex can become a source of isolation and criticism.

For avoiding complexities, adolescents must be brought up with a sense of equality for all. This is possible only if parents and elders set a proper example before them.

Evil Company

Bad Company is the source of all evil and atrocities. Bad friends are worse than the bitterest enemies. Adolescents learn most things from their friends. If they are not good, habits such as smoking, drugs, drinking or gambling can be learnt. Parents must be completely aware about the kind of friends or company their children keep. There should be no compromise in this regard. Bad Company can ruin the life of an individual. This holds good for persons of all ages.

To remove the above problems, it is necessary to divert the interests of the adolescent towards constructive ends. Students, who are shy, need to be exposed to debating, speaking and singing. Those who suffer from inferiority complex need to develop certain skills that can make them develop their cutting edge over others. Evil company can be avoided only when an adolescent is exposed to good books, a congenial family atmosphere and the inculcation of productive hobbies such as gardening, reading, playing musical instruments etc.

But the greatest problem that confronts an adolescent is to match his desires with the desires of his parents. The difficulty actually arises if John wants to become a writer but his parents want him to become an engineer. Such confrontations give rise to frustrations, depression and stress.

Many great men and women have been confronted by similar situations, but they could find an answer to them.

Always a Winner

There are some people in the world who are **Born to win**. Their mental courage and confidence always make them face every storm. Although they may fail in one task or another, their greatness continues to live even after their death. Nothing comes in the path of their mission. Neither the barrier of age, nor of sex, colour, creed, caste or wealth. One such Person who almost stands apart in the history of Britain is **Horatio Nelson**.

Horatio Nelson - The Born Winner

The entire way was filled with snow and it was almost dangerous to travel through the wild paths of eighteenth century Norfolk. The way was a narrow road across a marshland. A young boy of twelve was going to school with his brother William. They were asked to return home because walking in the snow could prove fatal. The young boy refused to return. His honour was at stake. He preferred death to retreat. He continued moving forward. They finally reached the deep drifts of snow which made their way extremely difficult. William thought it safe to return. But his brother simply refused. "We must go on", he said, "remember, it was left to our honour." That boy eventually reached home with his brother William. When his grandmother enquired whether he was fearful, he asked "What is fear?" The boy was none other than Horatio Nelson.

Horatio Nelson was the sixth member in a family of eleven. He was a sickly child. But he possessed unparalleled mental strength. His father was a country priest and his mother was a very pious lady. His parents were extremely poor. When he was hardly nine years old, his mother died. At the tender age of twelve he joined the Navy when cruelty, intoxication, whipping, revolt and murder were the regular features of Sea-life.

Nelson was so poor and weak that people thought that he would perish at sea. However, he succeeded in overcoming his physical weakness merely by determination. He never wanted to lose any task he undertook. And even if he did, he never accepted defeat mentally. He did those things which others never dared to do. Once he stole some apples from a garden and gave them to his friends saying that he did so because others were afraid to do so. In this attitude lies the secret of Nelson's greatness–to do what others do not dare to do.

Nelson always possessed a keen desire to be adventurous. He managed to get himself appointed in the ship Seahorse, which was proceeding towards the East Indies but within two years he became seriously ill and was compelled to return home. Ill-health brought him severe depression. Nelson became thoroughly despondent. He was undergoing a severe mental crisis when all of a sudden, out of his mental agony, a fire was kindled within.

He took a vow of dedicating his life for his country and the King. "I will be a hero, and confiding in Providence, I will brave every danger."

That was the commencement of his journey towards greatness and self-confidence. Many a time he moved into the jaws of death and weathered the gravest storms. His mental courage gave him the strength to shake the roots of death itself.

Nelson, who was once a frail boy became a great Admiral. He went through the tough school of experiences and finally emerged victorious, but he always remained soft from within. He was always warm and generous; he never forgot the hardships that he faced and always inspired his junior officers. He never forgot his friends, never ceased to exhibit compassion. Whenever he had any opportunity, he would always help others. And above all he was filled with glowing patriotism, an unfathomable desire to do his best for his country, England.

❑❑

Chapter Three

Strategy for Building Confidence

What is a Cybernetic Strategy?

Cybernetic Strategy is nothing but proper streamlined approach for undertaking any given task.

Like a war is always won with the help of a properly laid out plan, in the same way any work has to be done with the help of a carefully laid out plan. Similarly, to achieve greatness and nurturing confidence one has to carefully work out the strategy that can almost become a self-propellant for the achievement of success.

As a warrior, a person opting for greatness needs to answer the following questions?

- *What is my target?*
- *What are the major threats?*
- *How to approach the target?*
- *What is the strength of my army?*
- *In how much time do I have to capture the enemy territory?*
- *How will I be able to maintain my victory?*

So, the first step is none other than fixing the priorities.

Prioritizing

Every person has to fulfil various needs in life. These needs can be pertaining to the family, education, career or society. The various needs can be earning a livelihood, taking care of family, maintaining a social image, protest and success and spiritual development etc.

Maslow's theory says that a person first fulfils his physical needs such as food, clothing and shelter, after which he caters to his social needs such as success, name and fame and in the end his spiritual or moral needs. But history bears testimony to the fact that most of the great people dared to break this theory of Maslow's hierarchy and proceeded to set their own priorities. Great spiritual reformers have sacrificed their personal comforts, family and even food and shelter to seek God. They have focused their entire energies on a single priority - to attain divinity! And in spite of all the odds, they have startled mankind by attaining the heights of spiritual powers which was almost inconceivable for the majority of mankind. They have taught to the world to set priorities according to one's strong will and not according to conventional systems, which an average person tends to follow with the fear of social dogmas.

Here, we shall meet a spiritual giant whose priority was to liberate himself and his fellow brethren from sorrow. His name was Siddhartha, later acclaimed as Gautam Buddha.

Gautam Buddha

The entire kingdom was rejoicing the birth of a prince. The palace was overflowing with riches and pleasure. The king and the queen were doting upon the child. But the child's father was lost in his thoughts. He was deeply moved to see the suffering of mankind. Of what use was a son to him who would also be subjected to the old age, disease and death. Why was the life of man subjected to suffering? His mind was violently turbulent in search of truth. And at the dead of night when all retired he rose silently. He saw his little son peacefully resting in the arms of his beautiful wife. He felt a burning urge to clasp the baby in his arms. He managed to curb his impulses. But had he come to the world to be tied down by family ties or was he destined to search enlightenment not only for himself but for the entire humanity? Leaving all the comforts and pleasures behind him, he set out in search of the Eternal Truth. His priority in life was the quest for Spiritual Truth.

Gautam Buddha began his wanderings across the fertile plains of Ganges till he reached the land in the South. He lived there for six years subjecting himself to rigorous penance and asceticism. He shaved off his head, adorned his body with yellow robes and subjected his body to severe fasts and every recognized form of physical penance. He lived in a forest along with five disciples, exerting through self-discipline the mission of attaining truth.

He came to be known as a pious man, yet he was still oblivious of Truth. His priority in life was not recognition or settling down for mental peace, but to unravel the ultimate spiritual truths. One day, on waking up from a fainting fit produced by his extreme asceticism, a flashing light appeared before his eyes. He realized that physical mortification or extreme fasting was leading him nowhere. He felt the need of preserving his body for achieving his goal. Exhilarated by his realization and a hope for further accomplishments, Gautam wandered through the forests of Gaya in Bihar.

And finally after abiding hour upon hour of splintering mental and spiritual distress, after ranging through every feeling and emotion known to man, from the darkest despair to the brightest hope, Gautam found at last the mission of his life. He became Buddha - the Enlightened One.

He carried out his relentless work against Human suffering and established one of the greatest religions of the world. He ultimately accomplished what he had set his heart to. What he possessed was an unwavering devotion and self-confidence towards his mission.

Planning

Organizing

People who have accomplished Great missions in Life have always been great organizers. They carefully work on the art of motivating and managing people. People who have failed to manage armies, teams or groups have ended up with failures in life. The greatness of a person lies not in moving alone but in carrying along with him people of different mental frame-work. An able organizer always possesses the following qualities:

Tactful

An organizer must be very careful in dealing with colleagues and also subordinates. It is extremely important to keep one's temper mild and be very choosy with words. Harsh words can cause injury not only to personal relationships but also to business dealings. If there is any problem within the organization, it must be nipped in the bud by calling everybody across the table and discussing matters at length. But any sort of rudeness must be avoided as far as possible.

Decision maker

A good organizer is always a prompt decision-maker. He never waits upon crucial decisions for a very long time, rather acts at the right time. An organizer must know what to decide, when to decide, how to decide and most importantly in whose favour to decide. Delays in making decisions can bring losses to an organization.

Manager of contradictions

Where there are several people working, there is bound to be clash of opinions. A good organizer must know how to manage contradictory ideas and persons without being partial. An organization has to consider every viewpoint before deriving conclusions. Moreover, he must remain cool and composed amidst contradictory opinions and should not lose his own equilibrium. Contradictions must be borne with until they are in the best interest of the organization but not beyond that.

Democratic

A good organizer never imposes his own viewpoint forcefully. He rather tries to give an opportunity to each person for exhibiting his talents. A tyrannical organizer cannot survive for a very long time and even if he somehow survives, can never win the admiration and respect of his team members.

Patient

A suitable organizer is extremely patient under all circumstances. If he fails to accomplish a particular task, he does not throw tantrums, rather reviews the entire work, analyses the drawbacks and remotivates the people for further action. He always pursues a task till its successful completion, knows how to keep the adrenaline of his people high.

Receptive

An organizer is always receptive to novel ideas. He keeps himself charged and abreast with changing trends and tries to accommodate his tasks according to the times. He does not keep his mind in a water-tight compartment rather allows the free flow of ideas from all quarters. He is never hesitant to adopt changes and ideas even from subordinates.

Time Scheduling

Apart from organizing, time scheduling is another significant aspect for ensuring success. There is a very old proverb saying "Time and tide wait for no man". Time never waits for man, it is man who has to wait for the right time for doing a work. Man does not know what will happen to him in future. Hence, he has to live every moment to its full.

If you are speeding yourself towards greatness, you must learn the art of proper scheduling.

Prepare weekly schedules for yourself. The schedule must be on the basis of work and not on the basis of time. For example, if you are a student preparing for an examination, you must make up your mind that in one week you have to thoroughly complete three chapters of a particular subject and two of another. On the other hand, if you assign 3.00 p.m to 5.00 p.m for studies but at the end of the week, end up with preparing hardly a couple of chapters, your scheduling will prove to be futile. Hence scheduling must always be task based.

The Significance of Motivation

Apart from a proper management of systems, it is also very necessary to motivate and develop a good temperament.

Every person in this world has a different temperament, a different level of motivation and a different psyche. Therefore, a good organizer or a team leader must be fully conversant with the psyche of his team members and know how to boost their spirits during crisis.

There are mainly two kinds of motivations.

Positive

Positive motivation is meant for all those who possess a soft temperament, especially children and females. It must be adopted by those people who have a predominance of virtues and can be easily motivated. They should be charged with a strong mission, with incentives and accolades. They must be provided help whenever necessary and in times of crisis, they must resort to consoling and inspiring words. Such people can perform better under pressure. If you regard yourself as one among those, you must seek a noble teacher, a loyal friend and motivating books. This will help you to reaffirm your strength.

Negative

The second kind of motivation which at certain times can be dangerous is suitable for those people who have evil propensities. They are always attracted towards evil. If their pride is wounded and given a proper direction, they can produce wonders. Those who have negative attributes have greater strength to make it big, provided their energies can be fruitfully harnessed. It was easier for Dacoit Valmiki to become a Saint because of the possession of great strength. Negative motivation can include mild punishments or isolation that can make a person realize. However, it can also be dangerous in some cases, especially with children.

Failure or humiliation has also worked as a motivating factor for many people. The renowned poet Kalidas was one of those, who after facing humiliation from his wife, set out on the path of great learning.

Motivation can, however, lead to success only when one learns how to overcome hurdles.

❑❑

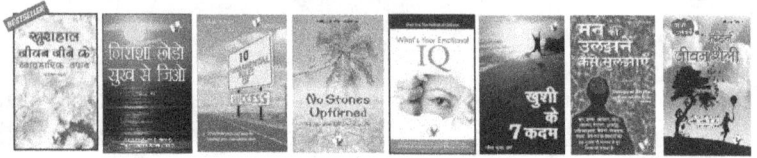

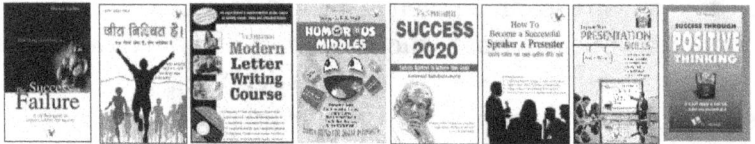

Also Available
in Hindi

Also Available
in Hindi

Also Available
in Kannada, Tamil

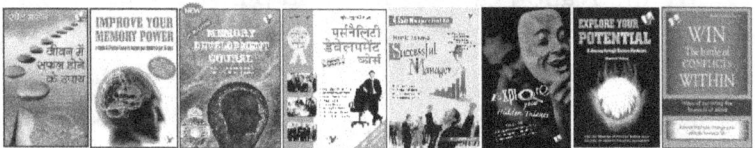

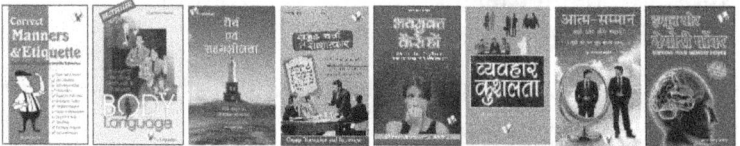

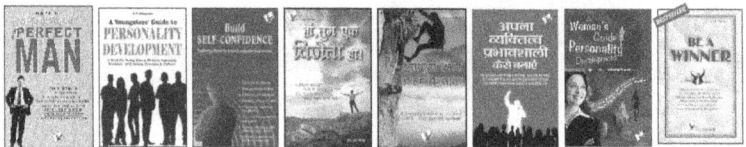

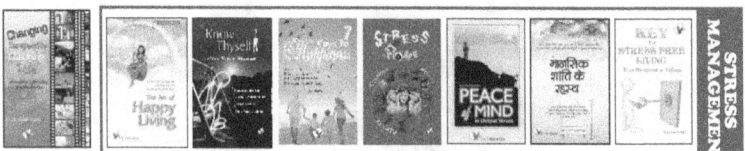

Also Available
in Kannada

Also Available
in Kannada

STRESS MANAGEMEN

All books available at www.vspublishers.com

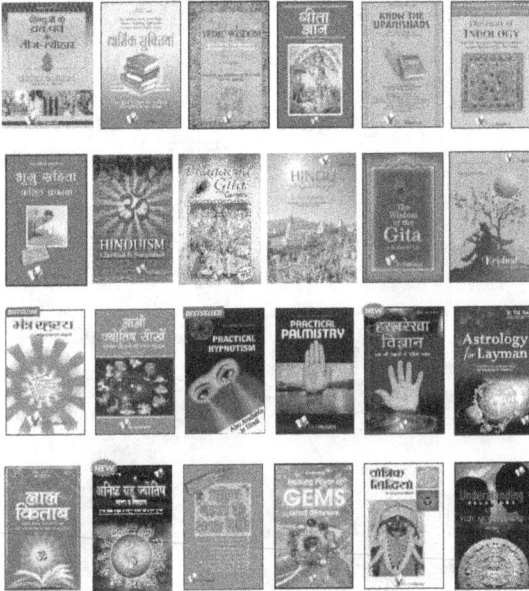

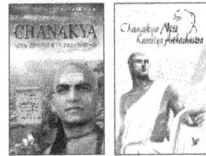

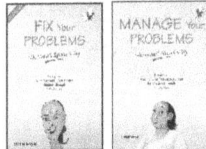

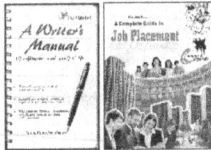

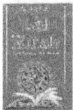

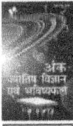

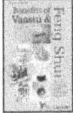

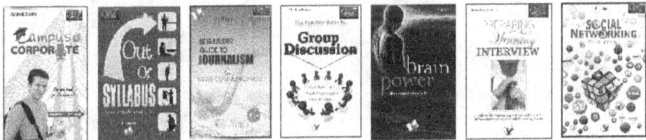

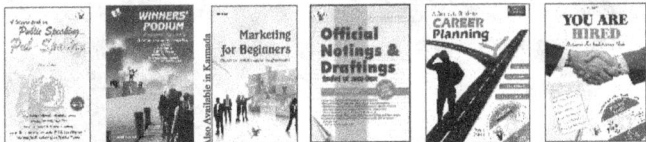

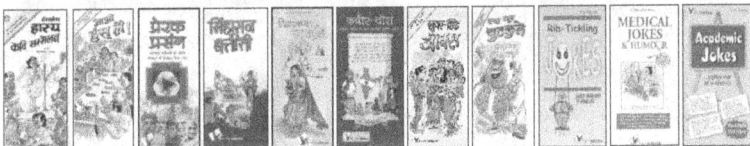

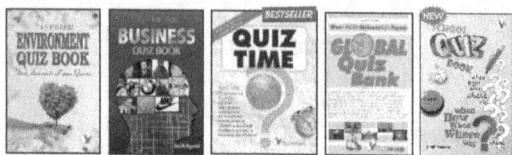

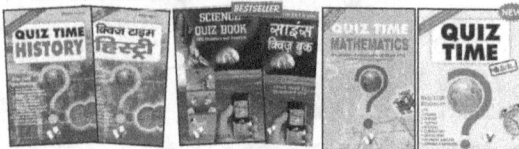

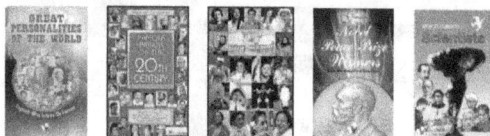

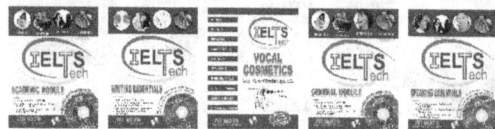

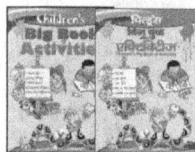

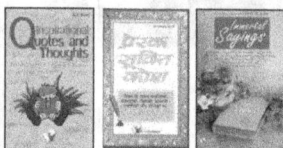

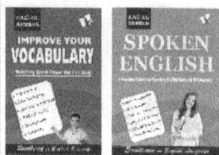

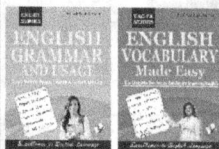

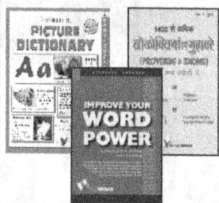

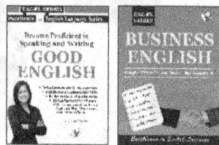

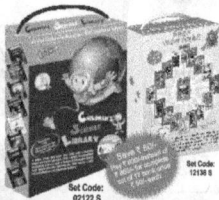

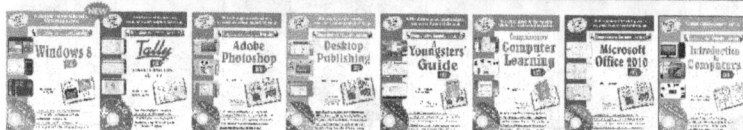

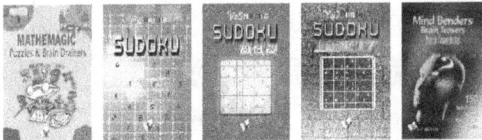

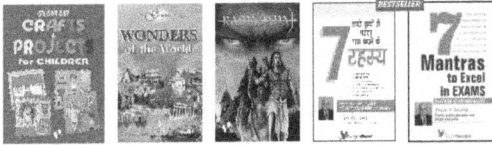

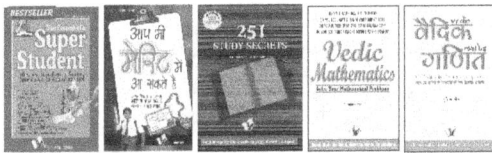

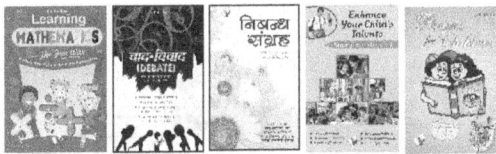

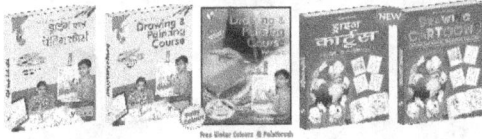

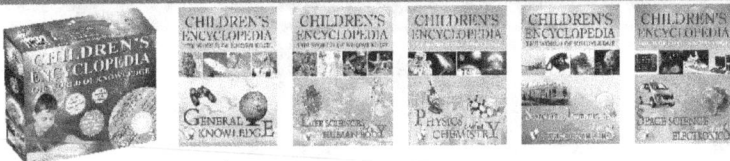

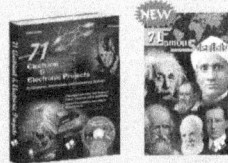

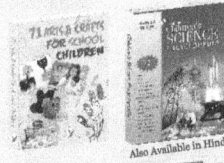

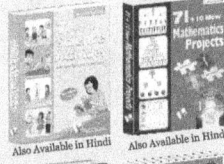

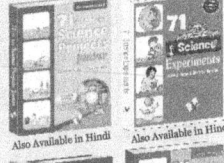

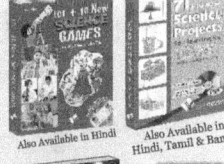

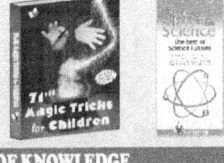

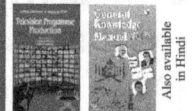

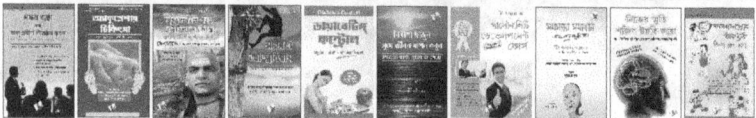

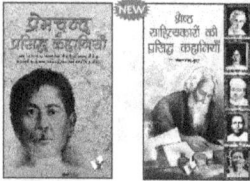

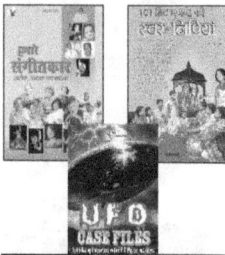

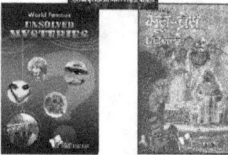

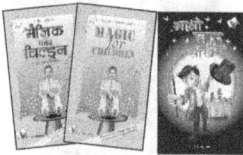

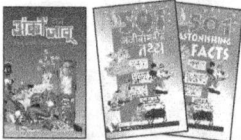

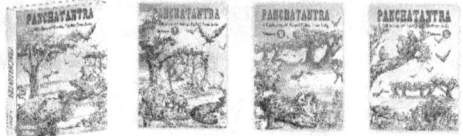

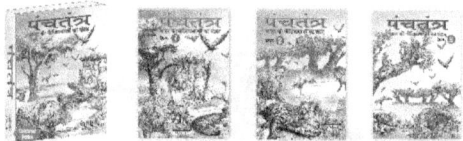

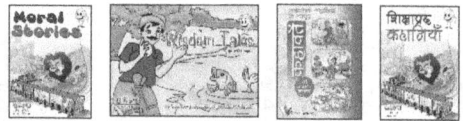

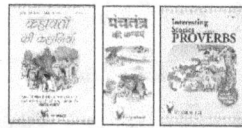

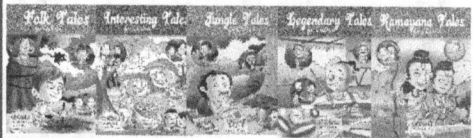

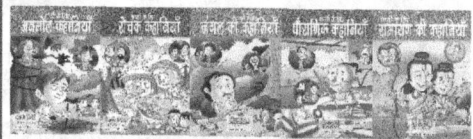